WEEK 1

WEEK BEGINNING:

CURRENT WEIGHT:

EXCITED?

You got this.

DATE   **DAY #**

BREAKFAST   FAT   PRTN CARB

                                                       CALS:

LUNCH   FAT   PRTN CARB

                                                       CALS:

DINNER   FAT   PRTN CARB

                                                       CALS:

SNACKS   FAT   PRTN CARB

                                                       CALS:

NOTES: **TOTALS**
                                                       FAT   PRTN CARB

I DRANK   **WATER**   **GOALS**
MY **PEE** WAS   FAT   PRTN CARB
I HAD   **ENERGY**
MY **MENTAL CLARITY** WAS
I **SLEPT**   HOURS AND FELT
MY **EXERCISE** WAS
AND I DID IT FOR   MINUTES AND FELT

DATE ______________________ DAY # ______________________

START WEIGHT: ___________ NOW WEIGHT: ___________ GOAL WEIGHT: ___________

CURRENT MOTIVATIONS: ______________________
____
____
____

CURRENT SUCCESSES: ______________________
____
____
____

LEARNING CURVES: ______________________
____
____
____

NEXT WEEK'S PLAN: ______________________
____
____
____

DATE   **DAY #**

BREAKFAST   FAT   PRTN CARB

                                                           CALS:

LUNCH   FAT   PRTN CARB

                                                           CALS:

DINNER   FAT   PRTN CARB

                                                           CALS:

SNACKS   FAT   PRTN CARB

                                                           CALS:

NOTES: **TOTALS**
                                                           FAT   PRTN CARB

                                                           GOALS
I DRANK ________________ **WATER**   FAT   PRTN CARB
MY **PEE** WAS ________________
I HAD ________________ **ENERGY**
MY **MENTAL CLARITY** WAS ________________
I **SLEPT** ________ HOURS AND FELT ________________
MY **EXERCISE** WAS ________________
AND I DID IT FOR ________ MINUTES AND FELT ________________

DATE   DAY #

START WEIGHT: NOW WEIGHT: GOAL WEIGHT:

CURRENT MOTIVATIONS: ______________________
____
____
____

CURRENT SUCCESSES: ______________________
____
____
____

LEARNING CURVES: ______________________
____
____
____

NEXT WEEK'S PLAN: ______________________
____
____
____

DATE   **DAY #**

BREAKFAST   FAT   PRTN CARB

                                                CALS:

LUNCH   FAT   PRTN CARB

                                                CALS:

DINNER   FAT   PRTN CARB

                                                CALS:

SNACKS   FAT   PRTN CARB

                                                CALS:

                                                TOTALS
NOTES: FAT   PRTN CARB

                                                GOALS
I DRANK _______________ **WATER**   FAT   PRTN CARB
MY **PEE** WAS _______________
I HAD _______________ **ENERGY**
MY **MENTAL CLARITY** WAS _______________
I **SLEPT** _____ HOURS AND FELT _______________
MY **EXERCISE** WAS _______________
AND I DID IT FOR _____ MINUTES AND FELT _______________

DATE   DAY #

START WEIGHT: NOW WEIGHT: GOAL WEIGHT:

CURRENT MOTIVATIONS: ______________________
____
____
____

CURRENT SUCCESSES: ______________________
____
____
____

LEARNING CURVES: ______________________
____
____
____

NEXT WEEK'S PLAN: ______________________
____
____
____

DATE   DAY #

BREAKFAST   FAT   PRTN CARB

                                                       CALS:

LUNCH   FAT   PRTN CARB

                                                       CALS:

DINNER   FAT   PRTN CARB

                                                       CALS:

SNACKS   FAT   PRTN CARB

                                                       CALS:

NOTES: **TOTALS**
                                                       FAT   PRTN CARB

                                                       GOALS
I DRANK _____________________ **WATER**   FAT   PRTN CARB
MY **PEE** WAS _______________
I HAD _______________ **ENERGY**
MY **MENTAL CLARITY** WAS _______________
I **SLEPT** _______ HOURS AND FELT _______________
MY **EXERCISE** WAS _______________
AND I DID IT FOR _______ MINUTES AND FELT _______________

CURRENT MOTIVATIONS: ___________________
____
____
____

CURRENT SUCCESSES: ___________________
____
____
____

LEARNING CURVES: ___________________
____
____
____

NEXT WEEK'S PLAN: ___________________
____
____
____

DATE   **DAY #**

BREAKFAST   FAT   PRTN CARB

                                                                CALS:

LUNCH   FAT   PRTN CARB

                                                                CALS:

DINNER   FAT   PRTN CARB

                                                                CALS:

SNACKS   FAT   PRTN CARB

                                                                CALS:

NOTES: **TOTALS**
                                                    FAT   PRTN CARB

I DRANK ________________ **WATER**   **GOALS**
MY **PEE** WAS ___________   FAT   PRTN CARB
I HAD ________________ **ENERGY**
MY **MENTAL CLARITY** WAS ___________
I **SLEPT** _______ HOURS AND FELT ___________
MY **EXERCISE** WAS ___________
AND I DID IT FOR _______ MINUTES AND FELT ___________

DATE   DAY #

START WEIGHT: NOW WEIGHT: GOAL WEIGHT:

CURRENT MOTIVATIONS: ___________________
____
____
____

CURRENT SUCCESSES: ___________________
____
____
____

LEARNING CURVES: ___________________
____
____
____

NEXT WEEK'S PLAN: ___________________
____
____

DATE   DAY #

BREAKFAST   FAT   PRTN CARB

                                              CALS:

LUNCH   FAT   PRTN CARB

                                              CALS:

DINNER   FAT   PRTN CARB

                                              CALS:

SNACKS   FAT   PRTN CARB

                                              CALS:

NOTES: **TOTALS**
                                              FAT   PRTN CARB

I DRANK _________________ **WATER**   **GOALS**
MY **PEE** WAS   FAT   PRTN CARB
I HAD _________________ **ENERGY**
MY **MENTAL CLARITY** WAS
I **SLEPT** _____ HOURS AND FELT
MY **EXERCISE** WAS
AND I DID IT FOR _____ MINUTES AND FELT

DATE   DAY #

START WEIGHT: NOW WEIGHT: GOAL WEIGHT:

CURRENT MOTIVATIONS: _______________

____

____

____

CURRENT SUCCESSES: _______________

____

____

____

LEARNING CURVES: _______________

____

____

____

NEXT WEEK'S PLAN: _______________

____

____

____

DATE   **DAY #**

BREAKFAST   FAT   PRTN   CARB

                                            CALS:

LUNCH   FAT   PRTN   CARB

                                            CALS:

DINNER   FAT   PRTN   CARB

                                            CALS:

SNACKS   FAT   PRTN   CARB

                                            CALS:

NOTES: **TOTALS**
                                            FAT   PRTN   CARB

I DRANK _______________ **WATER**   **GOALS**
MY **PEE** WAS   FAT   PRTN   CARB
I HAD _______________ **ENERGY**
MY **MENTAL CLARITY** WAS
I **SLEPT** _______ HOURS AND FELT
MY **EXERCISE** WAS
AND I DID IT FOR _______ MINUTES AND FELT

DATE   DAY #

START WEIGHT: NOW WEIGHT: GOAL WEIGHT:

CURRENT MOTIVATIONS: ________________

____

____

____

CURRENT SUCCESSES: ________________

____

____

____

LEARNING CURVES: ________________

____

____

____

NEXT WEEK'S PLAN: ________________

____

____

____

WEEK 2

WEEK BEGINNING: CURRENT WEIGHT:

HOW'S IT GOING?

You're killing at this!

DATE   **DAY #**

BREAKFAST   FAT   PRTN CARB

CALS:

LUNCH   FAT   PRTN CARB

CALS:

DINNER   FAT   PRTN CARB

CALS:

SNACKS   FAT   PRTN CARB

CALS:

NOTES:

TOTALS

FAT   PRTN CARB

GOALS

FAT   PRTN CARB

I DRANK __________________ **WATER**

MY **PEE** WAS __________________

I HAD __________________ **ENERGY**

MY **MENTAL CLARITY** WAS __________________

I **SLEPT** __________ HOURS AND FELT __________

MY **EXERCISE** WAS __________________

AND I DID IT FOR __________ MINUTES AND FELT __________

CURRENT MOTIVATIONS: _______________
____
____
____

CURRENT SUCCESSES: _______________
____
____
____

LEARNING CURVES: _______________
____
____
____

NEXT WEEK'S PLAN: _______________
____
____
____

DATE   **DAY #**

BREAKFAST   FAT PRTN CARB

                                            CALS:

LUNCH   FAT PRTN CARB

                                            CALS:

DINNER   FAT PRTN CARB

                                            CALS:

SNACKS   FAT PRTN CARB

                                            CALS:

NOTES: **TOTALS**
                                            FAT PRTN CARB

                                            GOALS
I DRANK   **WATER**   FAT PRTN CARB

MY **PEE** WAS

I HAD   **ENERGY**

MY **MENTAL CLARITY** WAS

I **SLEPT**   HOURS AND FELT

MY **EXERCISE** WAS

AND I DID IT FOR   MINUTES AND FELT

DATE   DAY #

START WEIGHT: NOW WEIGHT: GOAL WEIGHT:

CURRENT MOTIVATIONS: ______________________

____

____

____

CURRENT SUCCESSES: ______________________

____

____

____

LEARNING CURVES: ______________________

____

____

____

NEXT WEEK'S PLAN: ______________________

____

____

____

DATE   **DAY #**

BREAKFAST   FAT   PRTN CARB

                                                     CALS:

LUNCH   FAT   PRTN CARB

                                                     CALS:

DINNER   FAT   PRTN CARB

                                                     CALS:

SNACKS   FAT   PRTN CARB

                                                     CALS:

NOTES: **TOTALS**
                                             FAT   PRTN CARB

I DRANK _____________ **WATER**   **GOALS**
MY **PEE** WAS   FAT   PRTN CARB
I HAD _____________ **ENERGY**
MY **MENTAL CLARITY** WAS _____________
I **SLEPT** _____ HOURS AND FELT _____________
MY **EXERCISE** WAS _____________
AND I DID IT FOR _____ MINUTES AND FELT _____________

DATE   **DAY #**

START WEIGHT: **NOW WEIGHT:**   **GOAL WEIGHT:**

CURRENT MOTIVATIONS: ______________

____

____

____

CURRENT SUCCESSES: ______________

____

____

____

LEARNING CURVES: ______________

____

____

____

NEXT WEEK'S PLAN: ______________

____

____

____

DATE   DAY #

BREAKFAST   FAT   PRTN CARB

                                          CALS:

LUNCH   FAT   PRTN CARB

                                          CALS:

DINNER   FAT   PRTN CARB

                                          CALS:

SNACKS   FAT   PRTN CARB

                                          CALS:

NOTES: **TOTALS**
                                          FAT   PRTN CARB

I DRANK   **WATER**   **GOALS**
MY **PEE** WAS   FAT   PRTN CARB
I HAD   **ENERGY**
MY **MENTAL CLARITY** WAS
I **SLEPT**   HOURS AND FELT
MY **EXERCISE** WAS
AND I DID IT FOR   MINUTES AND FELT

DATE   **DAY #**

START WEIGHT: **NOW WEIGHT:**   **GOAL WEIGHT:**

CURRENT MOTIVATIONS: _______________

____

____

____

CURRENT SUCCESSES: _______________

____

____

____

LEARNING CURVES: _______________

____

____

____

NEXT WEEK'S PLAN: _______________

____

____

____

DATE   **DAY #**

BREAKFAST   FAT   PRTN CARB

                                                CALS:

LUNCH   FAT   PRTN CARB

                                                CALS:

DINNER   FAT   PRTN CARB

                                                CALS:

SNACKS   FAT   PRTN CARB

                                                CALS:

NOTES: **TOTALS**
                                                FAT   PRTN CARB

                                                GOALS
I DRANK   **WATER**   FAT   PRTN CARB

MY **PEE** WAS

I HAD   **ENERGY**

MY **MENTAL CLARITY** WAS

I **SLEPT**   HOURS AND FELT

MY **EXERCISE** WAS

AND I DID IT FOR   MINUTES AND FELT

CURRENT MOTIVATIONS: _______________

____

____

____

CURRENT SUCCESSES: _______________

____

____

____

LEARNING CURVES: _______________

____

____

____

NEXT WEEK'S PLAN: _______________

____

____

____

DATE   **DAY #**

BREAKFAST   FAT   PRTN   CARB

CALS:

LUNCH   FAT   PRTN   CARB

CALS:

DINNER   FAT   PRTN   CARB

CALS:

SNACKS   FAT   PRTN   CARB

CALS:

NOTES:

TOTALS

FAT   PRTN   CARB

GOALS

FAT   PRTN   CARB

I DRANK ________ **WATER**

MY **PEE** WAS ________

I HAD ________ **ENERGY**

MY **MENTAL CLARITY** WAS ________

I **SLEPT** ________ HOURS AND FELT ________

MY **EXERCISE** WAS ________

AND I DID IT FOR ________ MINUTES AND FELT ________

DATE ____________________ DAY # ____________

START WEIGHT: ________ NOW WEIGHT: ________ GOAL WEIGHT: ________

CURRENT MOTIVATIONS: ___________________
____
____
____

CURRENT SUCCESSES: ___________________
____
____
____

LEARNING CURVES: ___________________
____
____
____

NEXT WEEK'S PLAN: ___________________
____
____

DATE   DAY #

BREAKFAST   FAT   PRTN CARB

                                             CALS:

LUNCH   FAT   PRTN CARB

                                             CALS:

DINNER   FAT   PRTN CARB

                                             CALS:

SNACKS   FAT   PRTN CARB

                                             CALS:

NOTES: **TOTALS**
                                             FAT   PRTN CARB

I DRANK   WATER   **GOALS**
MY **PEE** WAS   FAT   PRTN CARB
I HAD   ENERGY
MY **MENTAL CLARITY** WAS
I **SLEPT**   HOURS AND FELT
MY **EXERCISE** WAS
AND I DID IT FOR   MINUTES AND FELT

CURRENT MOTIVATIONS: _________________

____

____

____

CURRENT SUCCESSES: _________________

____

____

____

LEARNING CURVES: _________________

____

____

____

NEXT WEEK'S PLAN: _________________

____

____

____

WEEK 3

WEEK BEGINNING: CURRENT WEIGHT:

HOW ARE YOU FEELING?

Your body loves you.

DATE   **DAY #**

BREAKFAST   FAT   PRTN CARB

CALS:

LUNCH   FAT   PRTN CARB

CALS:

DINNER   FAT   PRTN CARB

CALS:

SNACKS   FAT   PRTN CARB

CALS:

NOTES: **TOTALS**
                                                    FAT   PRTN CARB

I DRANK ______________ **WATER**   **GOALS**
MY **PEE** WAS   FAT   PRTN CARB
I HAD ______________ **ENERGY**
MY **MENTAL CLARITY** WAS
I **SLEPT** ______ HOURS AND FELT
MY **EXERCISE** WAS
AND I DID IT FOR ______ MINUTES AND FELT

CURRENT MOTIVATIONS: _______________

____

____

____

CURRENT SUCCESSES: _______________

____

____

____

LEARNING CURVES: _______________

____

____

____

NEXT WEEK'S PLAN: _______________

____

____

____

DATE   DAY #

BREAKFAST   FAT   PRTN CARB

                                         CALS:

LUNCH   FAT   PRTN CARB

                                         CALS:

DINNER   FAT   PRTN CARB

                                         CALS:

SNACKS   FAT   PRTN CARB

                                         CALS:

NOTES: **TOTALS**
                                         FAT   PRTN CARB

                                         GOALS
I DRANK   **WATER**   FAT   PRTN CARB
MY **PEE** WAS
I HAD   **ENERGY**
MY **MENTAL CLARITY** WAS
I **SLEPT**   HOURS AND FELT
MY **EXERCISE** WAS
AND I DID IT FOR   MINUTES AND FELT

DATE   DAY #

START WEIGHT: NOW WEIGHT: GOAL WEIGHT:

CURRENT MOTIVATIONS: ________________
____
____
____

CURRENT SUCCESSES: ________________
____
____
____

LEARNING CURVES: ________________
____
____
____

NEXT WEEK'S PLAN: ________________
____
____
____

DATE   DAY #

BREAKFAST   FAT   PRTN CARB

                                                   CALS:

LUNCH   FAT   PRTN CARB

                                                   CALS:

DINNER   FAT   PRTN CARB

                                                   CALS:

SNACKS   FAT   PRTN CARB

                                                   CALS:

NOTES: **TOTALS**
                                                   FAT   PRTN CARB

I DRANK   **WATER**   **GOALS**
MY **PEE** WAS   FAT   PRTN CARB
I HAD   **ENERGY**

MY **MENTAL CLARITY** WAS

I **SLEPT**   HOURS AND FELT

MY **EXERCISE** WAS

AND I DID IT FOR   MINUTES AND FELT

DATE   DAY #

START WEIGHT: NOW WEIGHT: GOAL WEIGHT:

CURRENT MOTIVATIONS: _______________________
____
____
____

CURRENT SUCCESSES: _________________________
____
____
____

LEARNING CURVES: ___________________________
____
____
____

NEXT WEEK'S PLAN: __________________________
____
____
____

DATE   **DAY #**

BREAKFAST   FAT   PRTN CARB

                                                      CALS:

LUNCH   FAT   PRTN CARB

                                                      CALS:

DINNER   FAT   PRTN CARB

                                                      CALS:

SNACKS   FAT   PRTN CARB

                                                      CALS:

NOTES: **TOTALS**
                                            FAT   PRTN CARB

GOALS
FAT   PRTN CARB

I DRANK ______________ **WATER**
MY **PEE** WAS
I HAD ______________ **ENERGY**
MY **MENTAL CLARITY** WAS
I **SLEPT** ______ HOURS AND FELT
MY **EXERCISE** WAS
AND I DID IT FOR ______ MINUTES AND FELT

DATE   DAY #

START WEIGHT: **NOW WEIGHT:**   **GOAL WEIGHT:**

CURRENT MOTIVATIONS: ______________

____

____

CURRENT SUCCESSES: ______________

____

____

LEARNING CURVES: ______________

____

____

NEXT WEEK'S PLAN: ______________

____

____

DATE   DAY #

BREAKFAST   FAT   PRTN CARB

                                             CALS:

LUNCH   FAT   PRTN CARB

                                             CALS:

DINNER   FAT   PRTN CARB

                                             CALS:

SNACKS   FAT   PRTN CARB

                                             CALS:

NOTES: **TOTALS**
                                             FAT   PRTN CARB

I DRANK   **WATER**   **GOALS**
MY **PEE** WAS   FAT   PRTN CARB
I HAD   **ENERGY**
MY **MENTAL CLARITY** WAS
I **SLEPT**   HOURS AND FELT
MY **EXERCISE** WAS
AND I DID IT FOR   MINUTES AND FELT

DATE   DAY #

START WEIGHT: NOW WEIGHT: GOAL WEIGHT:

CURRENT MOTIVATIONS: ______________________
____
____
____

CURRENT SUCCESSES: ______________________
____
____
____

LEARNING CURVES: ______________________
____
____
____

NEXT WEEK'S PLAN: ______________________
____
____
____

DATE   DAY #

BREAKFAST   FAT   PRTN   CARB

                                                CALS:

LUNCH   FAT   PRTN   CARB

                                                CALS:

DINNER   FAT   PRTN   CARB

                                                CALS:

SNACKS   FAT   PRTN   CARB

                                                CALS:

NOTES: **TOTALS**
                                                FAT   PRTN   CARB

I DRANK   **WATER**   **GOALS**
MY **PEE** WAS   FAT   PRTN   CARB
I HAD   **ENERGY**
MY **MENTAL CLARITY** WAS
I **SLEPT**   HOURS AND FELT
MY **EXERCISE** WAS
AND I DID IT FOR   MINUTES AND FELT

DATE   DAY #

START WEIGHT: NOW WEIGHT: GOAL WEIGHT:

CURRENT MOTIVATIONS: _______________

____

____

____

CURRENT SUCCESSES: _______________

____

____

____

LEARNING CURVES: _______________

____

____

____

NEXT WEEK'S PLAN: _______________

____

____

____

DATE   DAY #

BREAKFAST   FAT PRTN CARB

                                        CALS:

LUNCH   FAT PRTN CARB

                                        CALS:

DINNER   FAT PRTN CARB

                                        CALS:

SNACKS   FAT PRTN CARB

                                        CALS:

NOTES: **TOTALS**
                                        FAT PRTN CARB

I DRANK   **WATER**   **GOALS**
                                        FAT PRTN CARB
MY **PEE** WAS

I HAD   **ENERGY**

MY **MENTAL CLARITY** WAS

I **SLEPT**   HOURS AND FELT

MY **EXERCISE** WAS

AND I DID IT FOR   MINUTES AND FELT

DATE   DAY #

START WEIGHT: NOW WEIGHT: GOAL WEIGHT:

CURRENT MOTIVATIONS: ___________________
____
____
____

CURRENT SUCCESSES: ___________________
____
____
____

LEARNING CURVES: ___________________
____
____
____

NEXT WEEK'S PLAN: ___________________
____
____
____

WEEK 4

WEEK BEGINNING:

THINGS GOING WELL?

CURRENT WEIGHT:

The change in you is inspiring.

DATE   **DAY #**

BREAKFAST   FAT   PRTN CARB

                                      CALS:

LUNCH   FAT   PRTN CARB

                                      CALS:

DINNER   FAT   PRTN CARB

                                      CALS:

SNACKS   FAT   PRTN CARB

                                      CALS:

NOTES: **TOTALS**
                                      FAT   PRTN CARB

I DRANK   **WATER**   **GOALS**
MY **PEE** WAS   FAT   PRTN CARB
I HAD   **ENERGY**

MY **MENTAL CLARITY** WAS

I **SLEPT**   HOURS AND FELT

MY **EXERCISE** WAS

AND I DID IT FOR   MINUTES AND FELT

DATE   DAY #

START WEIGHT: NOW WEIGHT: GOAL WEIGHT:

CURRENT MOTIVATIONS: ___________________
____
____
____

CURRENT SUCCESSES: ___________________
____
____
____

LEARNING CURVES: ___________________
____
____
____

NEXT WEEK'S PLAN: ___________________
____
____
____

DATE   DAY #

BREAKFAST   FAT   PRTN   CARB

CALS:

LUNCH   FAT   PRTN   CARB

CALS:

DINNER   FAT   PRTN   CARB

CALS:

SNACKS   FAT   PRTN   CARB

CALS:

TOTALS

FAT   PRTN   CARB

NOTES:

GOALS

FAT   PRTN   CARB

I DRANK _______________ **WATER**

MY **PEE** WAS

I HAD _______________ **ENERGY**

MY **MENTAL CLARITY** WAS

I SLEPT _______ HOURS AND FELT

MY **EXERCISE** WAS

AND I DID IT FOR _______ MINUTES AND FELT

DATE   **DAY #**

START WEIGHT: **NOW WEIGHT:**   **GOAL WEIGHT:**

CURRENT MOTIVATIONS: ______________________

____

____

____

CURRENT SUCCESSES: ______________________

____

____

____

LEARNING CURVES: ______________________

____

____

____

NEXT WEEK'S PLAN: ______________________

____

____

____

DATE		DAY #		

BREAKFAST

FAT   PRTN   CARB

CALS:

LUNCH

FAT   PRTN   CARB

CALS:

DINNER

FAT   PRTN   CARB

CALS:

SNACKS

FAT   PRTN   CARB

CALS:

NOTES:

TOTALS		
FAT	PRTN	CARB

GOALS		
FAT	PRTN	CARB

I DRANK _______ **WATER**

MY **PEE** WAS

I HAD **ENERGY**

MY **MENTAL CLARITY** WAS

I **SLEPT** HOURS AND FELT

MY **EXERCISE** WAS

AND I DID IT FOR MINUTES AND FELT

DATE   DAY #

START WEIGHT: NOW WEIGHT: GOAL WEIGHT:

CURRENT MOTIVATIONS: ___________________

____

____

____

CURRENT SUCCESSES: ___________________

____

____

____

LEARNING CURVES: ___________________

____

____

____

NEXT WEEK'S PLAN: ___________________

____

____

____

DATE   **DAY #**

BREAKFAST   FAT   PRTN CARB

                                            CALS:

LUNCH   FAT   PRTN CARB

                                            CALS:

DINNER   FAT   PRTN CARB

                                            CALS:

SNACKS   FAT   PRTN CARB

                                            CALS:

NOTES: **TOTALS**
                                            FAT   PRTN CARB

I DRANK _______________ **WATER**   **GOALS**
MY **PEE** WAS _______________   FAT   PRTN CARB
I HAD _______________ **ENERGY**
MY **MENTAL CLARITY** WAS _______________
I **SLEPT** _______ HOURS AND FELT _______________
MY **EXERCISE** WAS _______________
AND I DID IT FOR _______ MINUTES AND FELT _______________

CURRENT MOTIVATIONS: __________________

____

____

____

CURRENT SUCCESSES: ___________________

____

____

____

LEARNING CURVES: _____________________

____

____

____

NEXT WEEK'S PLAN: ____________________

____

____

____

DATE   **DAY #**

BREAKFAST   FAT   PRTN CARB

                                            CALS:

LUNCH   FAT   PRTN CARB

                                            CALS:

DINNER   FAT   PRTN CARB

                                            CALS:

SNACKS   FAT   PRTN CARB

                                            CALS:

NOTES: **TOTALS**
                                            FAT   PRTN CARB

I DRANK _________________ **WATER**   **GOALS**
MY **PEE** WAS   FAT   PRTN CARB
I HAD _________________ **ENERGY**

MY **MENTAL CLARITY** WAS

I **SLEPT** _____ HOURS AND FELT

MY **EXERCISE** WAS

AND I DID IT FOR _____ MINUTES AND FELT

DATE   DAY #

START WEIGHT: NOW WEIGHT: GOAL WEIGHT:

CURRENT MOTIVATIONS: _______________
____
____
____

CURRENT SUCCESSES: _________________
____
____
____

LEARNING CURVES: ___________________
____
____
____

NEXT WEEK'S PLAN: __________________
____
____
____

DATE   **DAY #**

BREAKFAST   FAT   PRTN CARB

                                      CALS:

LUNCH   FAT   PRTN CARB

                                      CALS:

DINNER   FAT   PRTN CARB

                                      CALS:

SNACKS   FAT   PRTN CARB

                                      CALS:

NOTES: **TOTALS**
                                      FAT   PRTN CARB

I DRANK ________ **WATER**   **GOALS**
                                      FAT   PRTN CARB
MY **PEE** WAS

I HAD ________ **ENERGY**

MY **MENTAL CLARITY** WAS

I **SLEPT** ________ HOURS AND FELT

MY **EXERCISE** WAS

AND I DID IT FOR ________ MINUTES AND FELT

DATE   DAY #

START WEIGHT: NOW WEIGHT: GOAL WEIGHT:

CURRENT MOTIVATIONS: _______________

____

____

____

CURRENT SUCCESSES: _________________

____

____

____

LEARNING CURVES: ___________________

____

____

____

NEXT WEEK'S PLAN: ___________________

____

____

____

DATE   **DAY #**

BREAKFAST   FAT   PRTN CARB

CALS:

LUNCH   FAT   PRTN CARB

CALS:

DINNER   FAT   PRTN CARB

CALS:

SNACKS   FAT   PRTN CARB

CALS:

NOTES:

TOTALS
FAT   PRTN CARB

GOALS
FAT   PRTN CARB

I DRANK _______________ **WATER**
MY **PEE** WAS _______________
I HAD _______________ **ENERGY**
MY **MENTAL CLARITY** WAS _______________
I **SLEPT** _______ HOURS AND FELT _______
MY **EXERCISE** WAS _______________
AND I DID IT FOR _______ MINUTES AND FELT _______

CURRENT MOTIVATIONS: _______________
____
____
____

CURRENT SUCCESSES: _______________
____
____
____

LEARNING CURVES: _______________
____
____
____

NEXT WEEK'S PLAN: _______________
____
____
____

WEEK 5

WEEK BEGINNING: **CURRENT WEIGHT:**

ARE YOU ENJOYING THIS?

Keep calm and keto on!

DATE   **DAY #**

BREAKFAST   FAT   PRTN CARB

CALS:

LUNCH   FAT   PRTN CARB

CALS:

DINNER   FAT   PRTN CARB

CALS:

SNACKS   FAT   PRTN CARB

CALS:

NOTES: **TOTALS**
                                                    FAT   PRTN CARB

I DRANK ___________________ **WATER**   **GOALS**
MY **PEE** WAS ___________________   FAT   PRTN CARB
I HAD ___________________ **ENERGY**
MY **MENTAL CLARITY** WAS ___________________
I SLEPT ___________ HOURS AND FELT
MY **EXERCISE** WAS ___________________
AND I DID IT FOR ___________ MINUTES AND FELT

CURRENT MOTIVATIONS: ___________________

____

____

____

CURRENT SUCCESSES: ___________________

____

____

____

LEARNING CURVES: ___________________

____

____

____

NEXT WEEK'S PLAN: ___________________

____

____

____

DATE   **DAY #**

BREAKFAST   FAT   PRTN CARB

                                      CALS:

LUNCH   FAT   PRTN CARB

                                      CALS:

DINNER   FAT   PRTN CARB

                                      CALS:

SNACKS   FAT   PRTN CARB

                                      CALS:

NOTES: **TOTALS**
                                      FAT   PRTN CARB

                                      GOALS
I DRANK _______________ **WATER**   FAT   PRTN CARB
MY **PEE** WAS _______________
I HAD _______________ **ENERGY**

MY **MENTAL CLARITY** WAS _______________

I **SLEPT** ______ HOURS AND FELT _______________

MY **EXERCISE** WAS _______________

AND I DID IT FOR ______ MINUTES AND FELT _______________

CURRENT MOTIVATIONS: _______________
____
____
____

CURRENT SUCCESSES: _______________
____
____
____

LEARNING CURVES: _______________
____
____
____

NEXT WEEK'S PLAN: _______________
____
____
____

DATE   **DAY #**

BREAKFAST   FAT   PRTN CARB

                                                           CALS:

LUNCH   FAT   PRTN CARB

                                                           CALS:

DINNER   FAT   PRTN CARB

                                                           CALS:

SNACKS   FAT   PRTN CARB

                                                           CALS:

NOTES: **TOTALS**
                                                   FAT   PRTN CARB

I DRANK   **WATER**   **GOALS**
MY **PEE** WAS   FAT   PRTN CARB
I HAD   **ENERGY**
MY **MENTAL CLARITY** WAS
I **SLEPT**   HOURS AND FELT
MY **EXERCISE** WAS
AND I DID IT FOR   MINUTES AND FELT

DATE ___________________   DAY # ___________

START WEIGHT: __________ NOW WEIGHT: __________ GOAL WEIGHT: __________

CURRENT MOTIVATIONS: ________________________
____
____
____

CURRENT SUCCESSES: ________________________
____
____
____

LEARNING CURVES: ________________________
____
____
____

NEXT WEEK'S PLAN: ________________________
____
____
____

DATE   **DAY #**

BREAKFAST   FAT   PRTN CARB

                                            CALS:

LUNCH   FAT   PRTN CARB

                                            CALS:

DINNER   FAT   PRTN CARB

                                            CALS:

SNACKS   FAT   PRTN CARB

                                            CALS:

NOTES: **TOTALS**
                                            FAT   PRTN CARB

                                            GOALS
I DRANK ________________ **WATER**   FAT   PRTN CARB
MY **PEE** WAS ________________
I HAD ________________ **ENERGY**
MY **MENTAL CLARITY** WAS ________________
I **SLEPT** ______ HOURS AND FELT ________________
MY **EXERCISE** WAS ________________
AND I DID IT FOR ______ MINUTES AND FELT ________________

CURRENT MOTIVATIONS: ___________________

____

____

____

CURRENT SUCCESSES: ___________________

____

____

____

LEARNING CURVES: ___________________

____

____

____

NEXT WEEK'S PLAN: ___________________

____

____

____

DATE   **DAY #**

BREAKFAST   FAT   PRTN CARB

                                                 CALS:

LUNCH   FAT   PRTN CARB

                                                 CALS:

DINNER   FAT   PRTN CARB

                                                 CALS:

SNACKS   FAT   PRTN CARB

                                                 CALS:

NOTES: **TOTALS**
                                                 FAT   PRTN CARB

I DRANK ______________ **WATER**   **GOALS**
MY **PEE** WAS ______________   FAT   PRTN CARB
I HAD ______________ **ENERGY**
MY **MENTAL CLARITY** WAS ______________
I **SLEPT** ______ HOURS AND FELT
MY **EXERCISE** WAS ______________
AND I DID IT FOR ______ MINUTES AND FELT

CURRENT MOTIVATIONS: ___________________

____

____

____

CURRENT SUCCESSES: ___________________

____

____

____

LEARNING CURVES: ___________________

____

____

____

NEXT WEEK'S PLAN: ___________________

____

____

____

DATE   **DAY #**

BREAKFAST   FAT   PRTN CARB

                                               CALS:

LUNCH   FAT   PRTN CARB

                                               CALS:

DINNER   FAT   PRTN CARB

                                               CALS:

SNACKS   FAT   PRTN CARB

                                               CALS:

NOTES: **TOTALS**
                                            FAT   PRTN CARB

I DRANK ______________ **WATER**   **GOALS**
MY **PEE** WAS   FAT   PRTN CARB
I HAD ______________ **ENERGY**
MY **MENTAL CLARITY** WAS ______________
I **SLEPT** ______ HOURS AND FELT ______
MY **EXERCISE** WAS ______________
AND I DID IT FOR ______ MINUTES AND FELT ______

DATE   DAY #

START WEIGHT: NOW WEIGHT: GOAL WEIGHT:

CURRENT MOTIVATIONS: _______________

____

____

____

CURRENT SUCCESSES: _______________

____

____

____

LEARNING CURVES: _______________

____

____

____

NEXT WEEK'S PLAN: _______________

____

____

____

DATE   DAY #

BREAKFAST   FAT   PRTN CARB

                                                 CALS:

LUNCH   FAT   PRTN CARB

                                                 CALS:

DINNER   FAT   PRTN CARB

                                                 CALS:

SNACKS   FAT   PRTN CARB

                                                 CALS:

NOTES: **TOTALS**
                                                 FAT   PRTN CARB

                                          GOALS
I DRANK   **WATER**   FAT   PRTN CARB
MY **PEE** WAS
I HAD   **ENERGY**
MY **MENTAL CLARITY** WAS
I **SLEPT**   HOURS AND FELT
MY **EXERCISE** WAS
AND I DID IT FOR   MINUTES AND FELT

DATE   **DAY #**

START WEIGHT: **NOW WEIGHT:**   **GOAL WEIGHT:**

CURRENT MOTIVATIONS: ___________________________

____

____

____

CURRENT SUCCESSES: ___________________________

____

____

____

LEARNING CURVES: _____________________________

____

____

____

NEXT WEEK'S PLAN: _____________________________

____

____

____

WEEK 6

WEEK BEGINNING: CURRENT WEIGHT:

WHAT DIFFERENCES DO YOU SEE?

Already half way!

DATE   **DAY #**

BREAKFAST   FAT   PRTN CARB

                                                      CALS:

LUNCH   FAT   PRTN CARB

                                                      CALS:

DINNER   FAT   PRTN CARB

                                                      CALS:

SNACKS   FAT   PRTN CARB

                                                      CALS:

NOTES: **TOTALS**
                                                      FAT   PRTN CARB

I DRANK   **WATER**   **GOALS**
MY **PEE** WAS   FAT   PRTN CARB
I HAD   **ENERGY**

MY **MENTAL CLARITY** WAS
I SLEPT   HOURS AND FELT
MY **EXERCISE** WAS
AND I DID IT FOR   MINUTES AND FELT

DATE   **DAY #**

START WEIGHT: **NOW WEIGHT:**   **GOAL WEIGHT:**

CURRENT MOTIVATIONS: _______________________
____
____
____

CURRENT SUCCESSES: _______________________
____
____
____

LEARNING CURVES: _________________________
____
____
____

NEXT WEEK'S PLAN: ________________________
____
____
____

DATE   **DAY #**

BREAKFAST   FAT   PRTN CARB

CALS:

LUNCH   FAT   PRTN CARB

CALS:

DINNER   FAT   PRTN CARB

CALS:

SNACKS   FAT   PRTN CARB

CALS:

NOTES: **TOTALS**
                                                     FAT   PRTN CARB

I DRANK   **WATER**   **GOALS**
MY **PEE** WAS   FAT   PRTN CARB
I HAD   **ENERGY**
MY **MENTAL CLARITY** WAS
I **SLEPT**   HOURS AND FELT
MY **EXERCISE** WAS
AND I DID IT FOR   MINUTES AND FELT

DATE   **DAY #**

START WEIGHT: **NOW WEIGHT:**   **GOAL WEIGHT:**

CURRENT MOTIVATIONS: ___________________
____
____
____

CURRENT SUCCESSES: ___________________
____
____
____

LEARNING CURVES: ___________________
____
____
____

NEXT WEEK'S PLAN: ___________________
____
____
____

DATE   **DAY #**

BREAKFAST   FAT   PRTN CARB

                                                 CALS:

LUNCH   FAT   PRTN CARB

                                                 CALS:

DINNER   FAT   PRTN CARB

                                                 CALS:

SNACKS   FAT   PRTN CARB

                                                 CALS:

NOTES: **TOTALS**
                                        FAT   PRTN CARB

I DRANK   **WATER**   **GOALS**
MY **PEE** WAS   FAT   PRTN CARB
I HAD   **ENERGY**

MY **MENTAL CLARITY** WAS

I **SLEPT**   HOURS AND FELT

MY **EXERCISE** WAS

AND I DID IT FOR   MINUTES AND FELT

DATE   DAY #

START WEIGHT: _______   NOW WEIGHT: _______   GOAL WEIGHT: _______

CURRENT MOTIVATIONS: ______________________

____

____

____

CURRENT SUCCESSES: ______________________

____

____

____

LEARNING CURVES: ______________________

____

____

____

NEXT WEEK'S PLAN: ______________________

____

____

____

DATE   **DAY #**

BREAKFAST   FAT   PRTN CARB

                                                     CALS:

LUNCH   FAT   PRTN CARB

                                                     CALS:

DINNER   FAT   PRTN CARB

                                                     CALS:

SNACKS   FAT   PRTN CARB

                                                     CALS:

NOTES: **TOTALS**
                                                     FAT   PRTN CARB

I DRANK   **WATER**   **GOALS**
MY **PEE** WAS   FAT   PRTN CARB
I HAD   **ENERGY**

MY **MENTAL CLARITY** WAS

I SLEPT   HOURS AND FELT

MY **EXERCISE** WAS

AND I DID IT FOR   MINUTES AND FELT

DATE   **DAY #**

START WEIGHT: **NOW WEIGHT:**   **GOAL WEIGHT:**

CURRENT MOTIVATIONS: _______________
____
____
____

CURRENT SUCCESSES: _______________
____
____
____

LEARNING CURVES: _______________
____
____
____

NEXT WEEK'S PLAN: _______________
____
____

DATE   DAY #

BREAKFAST   FAT   PRTN   CARB

CALS:

LUNCH   FAT   PRTN   CARB

CALS:

DINNER   FAT   PRTN   CARB

CALS:

SNACKS   FAT   PRTN   CARB

CALS:

NOTES: **TOTALS**

FAT   PRTN   CARB

GOALS

FAT   PRTN   CARB

I DRANK   **WATER**

MY **PEE** WAS

I HAD   **ENERGY**

MY **MENTAL CLARITY** WAS

I SLEPT   HOURS AND FELT

MY **EXERCISE** WAS

AND I DID IT FOR   MINUTES AND FELT

DATE   **DAY #**

START WEIGHT: **NOW WEIGHT:**   **GOAL WEIGHT:**

CURRENT MOTIVATIONS: _______________________
____
____
____

CURRENT SUCCESSES: _______________________
____
____
____

LEARNING CURVES: _______________________
____
____
____

NEXT WEEK'S PLAN: _______________________
____
____

DATE   DAY #

BREAKFAST   FAT   PRTN CARB

                                                 CALS:

LUNCH   FAT   PRTN CARB

                                                 CALS:

DINNER   FAT   PRTN CARB

                                                 CALS:

SNACKS   FAT   PRTN CARB

                                                 CALS:

                                                 TOTALS
NOTES: FAT   PRTN CARB

                                                 GOALS
I DRANK   **WATER**   FAT   PRTN CARB
MY **PEE** WAS
I HAD   **ENERGY**
MY **MENTAL CLARITY** WAS
I **SLEPT**   HOURS AND FELT
MY **EXERCISE** WAS
AND I DID IT FOR   MINUTES AND FELT

CURRENT MOTIVATIONS: _______________

____

____

____

CURRENT SUCCESSES: _______________

____

____

____

LEARNING CURVES: _______________

____

____

____

NEXT WEEK'S PLAN: _______________

____

____

____

DATE   DAY #

BREAKFAST   FAT   PRTN CARB

CALS:

LUNCH   FAT   PRTN CARB

CALS:

DINNER   FAT   PRTN CARB

CALS:

SNACKS   FAT   PRTN CARB

CALS:

NOTES:

TOTALS

FAT   PRTN CARB

I DRANK   WATER

GOALS

FAT   PRTN CARB

MY **PEE** WAS

I HAD   ENERGY

MY **MENTAL CLARITY** WAS

I SLEPT   HOURS AND FELT

MY **EXERCISE** WAS

AND I DID IT FOR   MINUTES AND FELT

CURRENT MOTIVATIONS: ___________________
____
____
____

CURRENT SUCCESSES: ___________________
____
____
____

LEARNING CURVES: ___________________
____
____
____

NEXT WEEK'S PLAN: ___________________
____
____
____

WEEK 7

WEEK BEGINNING:

CURRENT WEIGHT:

FEELING GOOD?

Healthy tastes delicious.

DATE   DAY #

BREAKFAST   FAT   PRTN CARB

                                  CALS:

LUNCH   FAT   PRTN CARB

                                  CALS:

DINNER   FAT   PRTN CARB

                                  CALS:

SNACKS   FAT   PRTN CARB

                                  CALS:

                                  TOTALS
NOTES: FAT   PRTN CARB

                                  GOALS
I DRANK _______________ WATER   FAT   PRTN CARB
MY **PEE** WAS
I HAD ________________ ENERGY
MY **MENTAL CLARITY** WAS
I **SLEPT** ______ HOURS AND FELT
MY **EXERCISE** WAS
AND I DID IT FOR ______ MINUTES AND FELT

DATE   DAY #

START WEIGHT: NOW WEIGHT: GOAL WEIGHT:

CURRENT MOTIVATIONS: _______________

____

____

____

CURRENT SUCCESSES: _______________

____

____

____

LEARNING CURVES: _______________

____

____

____

NEXT WEEK'S PLAN: _______________

____

____

____

DATE   **DAY #**

BREAKFAST   FAT   PRTN CARB

                                                  CALS:

LUNCH   FAT   PRTN CARB

                                                  CALS:

DINNER   FAT   PRTN CARB

                                                  CALS:

SNACKS   FAT   PRTN CARB

                                                  CALS:

NOTES: **TOTALS**
                                                  FAT   PRTN CARB

I DRANK _______________ **WATER**   **GOALS**
MY **PEE** WAS _______________   FAT   PRTN CARB
I HAD _______________ **ENERGY**
MY **MENTAL CLARITY** WAS _______________
I **SLEPT** _______ HOURS AND FELT _______________
MY **EXERCISE** WAS _______________
AND I DID IT FOR _______ MINUTES AND FELT _______________

DATE   DAY #

START WEIGHT: NOW WEIGHT: GOAL WEIGHT:

CURRENT MOTIVATIONS: ______________

____

____

____

CURRENT SUCCESSES: ______________

____

____

____

LEARNING CURVES: ______________

____

____

____

NEXT WEEK'S PLAN: ______________

____

____

____

DATE   **DAY #**

BREAKFAST   FAT PRTN CARB

CALS:

LUNCH   FAT PRTN CARB

CALS:

DINNER   FAT PRTN CARB

CALS:

SNACKS   FAT PRTN CARB

CALS:

NOTES: **TOTALS**

FAT PRTN CARB

GOALS

FAT PRTN CARB

I DRANK   **WATER**

MY **PEE** WAS

I HAD   **ENERGY**

MY **MENTAL CLARITY** WAS

I **SLEPT**   HOURS AND FELT

MY **EXERCISE** WAS

AND I DID IT FOR   MINUTES AND FELT

DATE   DAY #

START WEIGHT: NOW WEIGHT: GOAL WEIGHT:

CURRENT MOTIVATIONS: ___________________
____
____
____

CURRENT SUCCESSES: _____________________
____
____
____

LEARNING CURVES: _______________________
____
____
____

NEXT WEEK'S PLAN: ______________________
____
____
____

DATE   **DAY #**

BREAKFAST   FAT   PRTN CARB

                                             CALS:

LUNCH   FAT   PRTN CARB

                                             CALS:

DINNER   FAT   PRTN CARB

                                             CALS:

SNACKS   FAT   PRTN CARB

                                             CALS:

NOTES: **TOTALS**
                                             FAT   PRTN CARB

I DRANK _____________ **WATER**   **GOALS**
MY **PEE** WAS _____________   FAT   PRTN CARB
I HAD _____________ **ENERGY**
MY **MENTAL CLARITY** WAS _____________
I **SLEPT** _____ HOURS AND FELT _____________
MY **EXERCISE** WAS _____________
AND I DID IT FOR _____ MINUTES AND FELT _____________

DATE   DAY #

START WEIGHT: NOW WEIGHT: GOAL WEIGHT:

CURRENT MOTIVATIONS: ___________________
____
____
____

CURRENT SUCCESSES: _____________________
____
____
____

LEARNING CURVES: _______________________
____
____
____

NEXT WEEK'S PLAN: _______________________
____
____
____

DATE   **DAY #**

BREAKFAST   FAT   PRTN CARB

                                          CALS:

LUNCH   FAT   PRTN CARB

                                          CALS:

DINNER   FAT   PRTN CARB

                                          CALS:

SNACKS   FAT   PRTN CARB

                                          CALS:

NOTES: **TOTALS**
                                          FAT   PRTN CARB

I DRANK _______________ **WATER**   **GOALS**
MY **PEE** WAS _______________   FAT   PRTN CARB
I HAD _______________ **ENERGY**

MY **MENTAL CLARITY** WAS _______________

I **SLEPT** _______ HOURS AND FELT _______________

MY **EXERCISE** WAS _______________

AND I DID IT FOR _______ MINUTES AND FELT _______________

DATE   DAY #

START WEIGHT: NOW WEIGHT: GOAL WEIGHT:

CURRENT MOTIVATIONS: ___________________
____
____
____

CURRENT SUCCESSES: ___________________
____
____
____

LEARNING CURVES: ___________________
____
____
____

NEXT WEEK'S PLAN: ___________________
____
____

DATE   **DAY #**

BREAKFAST   FAT   PRTN   CARB

                                           CALS:

LUNCH   FAT   PRTN   CARB

                                           CALS:

DINNER   FAT   PRTN   CARB

                                           CALS:

SNACKS   FAT   PRTN   CARB

                                           CALS:

NOTES: **TOTALS**
                                           FAT   PRTN   CARB

I DRANK   **WATER**   **GOALS**
MY **PEE** WAS   FAT   PRTN   CARB
I HAD   **ENERGY**
MY **MENTAL CLARITY** WAS
I **SLEPT**   HOURS AND FELT
MY **EXERCISE** WAS
AND I DID IT FOR   MINUTES AND FELT

CURRENT MOTIVATIONS: _______________________

____

____

____

CURRENT SUCCESSES: _______________________

____

____

____

LEARNING CURVES: _______________________

____

____

____

NEXT WEEK'S PLAN: _______________________

____

____

____

DATE

DAY #

BREAKFAST

FAT   PRTN   CARB

CALS:

LUNCH

FAT   PRTN   CARB

CALS:

DINNER

FAT   PRTN   CARB

CALS:

SNACKS

FAT   PRTN   CARB

CALS:

NOTES:

TOTALS

FAT   PRTN   CARB

GOALS

FAT   PRTN   CARB

I DRANK _____ **WATER**

MY **PEE** WAS _____

I HAD _____ **ENERGY**

MY **MENTAL CLARITY** WAS _____

I **SLEPT** _____ HOURS AND FELT _____

MY **EXERCISE** WAS _____

AND I DID IT FOR _____ MINUTES AND FELT _____

DATE   DAY #

START WEIGHT: NOW WEIGHT: GOAL WEIGHT:

CURRENT MOTIVATIONS: ________________
____
____
____

CURRENT SUCCESSES: ________________
____
____
____

LEARNING CURVES: ________________
____
____
____

NEXT WEEK'S PLAN: ________________
____
____
____

WEEK 8

WEEK BEGINNING: **CURRENT WEIGHT:**

FAVORITE KETO FOOD?

You're motivating people.

DATE   **DAY #**

BREAKFAST   FAT   PRTN CARB

                                           CALS:

LUNCH   FAT   PRTN CARB

                                           CALS:

DINNER   FAT   PRTN CARB

                                           CALS:

SNACKS   FAT   PRTN CARB

                                           CALS:

NOTES: **TOTALS**
                                           FAT   PRTN CARB

                                           GOALS
I DRANK _______________ **WATER**   FAT   PRTN CARB
MY **PEE** WAS _______________
I HAD _______________ **ENERGY**
MY **MENTAL CLARITY** WAS _______________
I **SLEPT** ______ HOURS AND FELT _______________
MY **EXERCISE** WAS _______________
AND I DID IT FOR ______ MINUTES AND FELT _______________

DATE _______________________ **DAY #** _______________________

START WEIGHT: _______ **NOW WEIGHT:** _______ **GOAL WEIGHT:** _______

CURRENT MOTIVATIONS: ____________________
____
____
____

CURRENT SUCCESSES: _____________________
____
____
____

LEARNING CURVES: ______________________
____
____
____

NEXT WEEK'S PLAN: ______________________
____
____
____

DATE   **DAY #**

BREAKFAST   FAT   PRTN   CARB

CALS:

LUNCH   FAT   PRTN   CARB

CALS:

DINNER   FAT   PRTN   CARB

CALS:

SNACKS   FAT   PRTN   CARB

CALS:

NOTES: **TOTALS**
                                      FAT   PRTN   CARB

I DRANK ________________ **WATER**   **GOALS**
MY **PEE** WAS ___________   FAT   PRTN   CARB
I HAD ___________ **ENERGY**
MY **MENTAL CLARITY** WAS __________
I **SLEPT** ______ HOURS AND FELT __________
MY **EXERCISE** WAS __________
AND I DID IT FOR ______ MINUTES AND FELT __________

DATE   DAY #

START WEIGHT: NOW WEIGHT: GOAL WEIGHT:

CURRENT MOTIVATIONS: ______________

____

____

____

CURRENT SUCCESSES: ______________

____

____

____

LEARNING CURVES: ______________

____

____

____

NEXT WEEK'S PLAN: ______________

____

____

____

DATE   **DAY #**

BREAKFAST   FAT   PRTN CARB

CALS:

LUNCH   FAT   PRTN CARB

CALS:

DINNER   FAT   PRTN CARB

CALS:

SNACKS   FAT   PRTN CARB

CALS:

NOTES: **TOTALS**

FAT   PRTN CARB

I DRANK ___________ **WATER**   **GOALS**

MY **PEE** WAS ___________   FAT   PRTN CARB

I HAD ___________ **ENERGY**

MY **MENTAL CLARITY** WAS ___________

I **SLEPT** ___________ HOURS AND FELT ___________

MY **EXERCISE** WAS ___________

AND I DID IT FOR ___________ MINUTES AND FELT ___________

DATE   DAY #

BREAKFAST   FAT   PRTN CARB

                                        CALS:

LUNCH   FAT   PRTN CARB

                                        CALS:

DINNER   FAT   PRTN CARB

                                        CALS:

SNACKS   FAT   PRTN CARB

                                        CALS:

NOTES: **TOTALS**
                                        FAT   PRTN CARB

GOALS
FAT   PRTN CARB

I DRANK   **WATER**
MY **PEE** WAS
I HAD   **ENERGY**
MY **MENTAL CLARITY** WAS
I **SLEPT**   HOURS AND FELT
MY **EXERCISE** WAS
AND I DID IT FOR   MINUTES AND FELT

CURRENT MOTIVATIONS: ___________________

____

____

____

CURRENT SUCCESSES: ___________________

____

____

____

LEARNING CURVES: ___________________

____

____

____

NEXT WEEK'S PLAN: ___________________

____

____

____

DATE   **DAY #**

BREAKFAST   FAT   PRTN CARB

CALS:

LUNCH   FAT   PRTN CARB

CALS:

DINNER   FAT   PRTN CARB

CALS:

SNACKS   FAT   PRTN CARB

CALS:

NOTES:

TOTALS

FAT   PRTN CARB

I DRANK   **WATER**

MY **PEE** WAS

I HAD   **ENERGY**

MY **MENTAL CLARITY** WAS

I **SLEPT**   HOURS AND FELT

MY **EXERCISE** WAS

AND I DID IT FOR   MINUTES AND FELT

GOALS

FAT   PRTN CARB

DATE   DAY #

START WEIGHT: NOW WEIGHT: GOAL WEIGHT:

CURRENT MOTIVATIONS: _______________
____
____
____

CURRENT SUCCESSES: _______________
____
____
____

LEARNING CURVES: _______________
____
____
____

NEXT WEEK'S PLAN: _______________
____
____
____

DATE   **DAY #**

BREAKFAST   FAT   PRTN CARB

                                             CALS:

LUNCH   FAT   PRTN CARB

                                             CALS:

DINNER   FAT   PRTN CARB

                                             CALS:

SNACKS   FAT   PRTN CARB

                                             CALS:

NOTES: **TOTALS**
                                             FAT   PRTN CARB

I DRANK _______________ **WATER**   **GOALS**
MY **PEE** WAS   FAT   PRTN CARB
I HAD _______________ **ENERGY**
MY **MENTAL CLARITY** WAS
I **SLEPT** _______ HOURS AND FELT
MY **EXERCISE** WAS
AND I DID IT FOR _______ MINUTES AND FELT

DATE   DAY #

START WEIGHT: NOW WEIGHT: GOAL WEIGHT:

CURRENT MOTIVATIONS: _______________
____
____
____

CURRENT SUCCESSES: _________________
____
____
____

LEARNING CURVES: ___________________
____
____
____

NEXT WEEK'S PLAN: ___________________
____
____

DATE   DAY #

BREAKFAST   FAT PRTN CARB

                                             CALS:

LUNCH   FAT PRTN CARB

                                             CALS:

DINNER   FAT PRTN CARB

                                             CALS:

SNACKS   FAT PRTN CARB

                                             CALS:

NOTES: **TOTALS**
                                             FAT PRTN CARB

                                             GOALS
I DRANK   **WATER**   FAT PRTN CARB
MY **PEE** WAS
I HAD   **ENERGY**
MY **MENTAL CLARITY** WAS
I **SLEPT**   HOURS AND FELT
MY **EXERCISE** WAS
AND I DID IT FOR   MINUTES AND FELT

CURRENT MOTIVATIONS: _______________
____
____
____

CURRENT SUCCESSES: _______________
____
____
____

LEARNING CURVES: _______________
____
____
____

NEXT WEEK'S PLAN: _______________
____
____
____

WEEK 9

WEEK BEGINNING: **CURRENT WEIGHT:**

CLOTHES FEELING LOOSER YET?

You're a natural at this.

DATE   DAY #

BREAKFAST   FAT   PRTN CARB

                                                    CALS:

LUNCH   FAT   PRTN CARB

                                                    CALS:

DINNER   FAT   PRTN CARB

                                                    CALS:

SNACKS   FAT   PRTN CARB

                                                    CALS:

NOTES: **TOTALS**
                                                    FAT   PRTN CARB

I DRANK _______________ **WATER**   **GOALS**
MY **PEE** WAS _______________   FAT   PRTN CARB
I HAD _______________ **ENERGY**
MY **MENTAL CLARITY** WAS _______________
I SLEPT _______ HOURS AND FELT _______________
MY **EXERCISE** WAS _______________
AND I DID IT FOR _______ MINUTES AND FELT _______________

DATE   DAY #

START WEIGHT: NOW WEIGHT: GOAL WEIGHT:

CURRENT MOTIVATIONS: __________________
____
____
____

CURRENT SUCCESSES: __________________
____
____
____

LEARNING CURVES: __________________
____
____
____

NEXT WEEK'S PLAN: __________________
____
____
____

DATE   **DAY #**

BREAKFAST   FAT   PRTN CARB

                                            CALS:

LUNCH   FAT   PRTN CARB

                                            CALS:

DINNER   FAT   PRTN CARB

                                            CALS:

SNACKS   FAT   PRTN CARB

                                            CALS:

NOTES: **TOTALS**
                                            FAT   PRTN CARB

I DRANK _______________ **WATER**   **GOALS**
MY **PEE** WAS   FAT   PRTN CARB
I HAD _______________ **ENERGY**
MY **MENTAL CLARITY** WAS
I **SLEPT** _____ HOURS AND FELT
MY **EXERCISE** WAS
AND I DID IT FOR _____ MINUTES AND FELT

DATE ______________________   DAY # ______________________

START WEIGHT: __________   NOW WEIGHT: __________   GOAL WEIGHT: __________

CURRENT MOTIVATIONS: _______________________

____

____

____

CURRENT SUCCESSES: _______________________

____

____

____

LEARNING CURVES: _______________________

____

____

____

NEXT WEEK'S PLAN: _______________________

____

____

____

DATE   **DAY #**

BREAKFAST   FAT   PRTN CARB

                                             CALS:

LUNCH   FAT   PRTN CARB

                                             CALS:

DINNER   FAT   PRTN CARB

                                             CALS:

SNACKS   FAT   PRTN CARB

                                             CALS:

NOTES: **TOTALS**
                                             FAT   PRTN CARB

I DRANK _______ **WATER**   **GOALS**
MY **PEE** WAS _______   FAT   PRTN CARB
I HAD _______ **ENERGY**
MY **MENTAL CLARITY** WAS _______
I **SLEPT** _______ HOURS AND FELT
MY **EXERCISE** WAS _______
AND I DID IT FOR _______ MINUTES AND FELT

DATE   DAY #

START WEIGHT: NOW WEIGHT: GOAL WEIGHT:

CURRENT MOTIVATIONS: _______________

____

____

____

CURRENT SUCCESSES: _______________

____

____

____

LEARNING CURVES: _______________

____

____

____

NEXT WEEK'S PLAN: _______________

____

____

DATE   **DAY #**

BREAKFAST   FAT   PRTN   CARB

                                                           CALS:

LUNCH   FAT   PRTN   CARB

                                                           CALS:

DINNER   FAT   PRTN   CARB

                                                           CALS:

SNACKS   FAT   PRTN   CARB

                                                           CALS:

NOTES: **TOTALS**
                                                   FAT   PRTN   CARB

                                                   GOALS
I DRANK ________________ **WATER**   FAT   PRTN   CARB

MY **PEE** WAS

I HAD ________________ **ENERGY**

MY **MENTAL CLARITY** WAS

I **SLEPT** ____ HOURS AND FELT

MY **EXERCISE** WAS

AND I DID IT FOR ____ MINUTES AND FELT

DATE   DAY #

START WEIGHT: NOW WEIGHT: GOAL WEIGHT:

CURRENT MOTIVATIONS: _______________

____

____

____

CURRENT SUCCESSES: _______________

____

____

____

LEARNING CURVES: _______________

____

____

____

NEXT WEEK'S PLAN: _______________

____

____

____

DATE   **DAY #**

BREAKFAST   FAT   PRTN CARB

                                                CALS:

LUNCH   FAT   PRTN CARB

                                                CALS:

DINNER   FAT   PRTN CARB

                                                CALS:

SNACKS   FAT   PRTN CARB

                                                CALS:

NOTES: **TOTALS**
                                                FAT   PRTN CARB

I DRANK ________________ **WATER**   **GOALS**
MY **PEE** WAS   FAT   PRTN CARB
I HAD ________________ **ENERGY**
MY **MENTAL CLARITY** WAS
I **SLEPT** ______ HOURS AND FELT
MY **EXERCISE** WAS
AND I DID IT FOR ______ MINUTES AND FELT

DATE   **DAY #**

START WEIGHT: **NOW WEIGHT:**   **GOAL WEIGHT:**

CURRENT MOTIVATIONS: _______________

____

____

____

CURRENT SUCCESSES: _______________

____

____

____

LEARNING CURVES: _______________

____

____

____

NEXT WEEK'S PLAN: _______________

____

____

____

DATE   **DAY #**

BREAKFAST   FAT   PRTN CARB

                                                     CALS:

LUNCH   FAT   PRTN CARB

                                                     CALS:

DINNER   FAT   PRTN CARB

                                                     CALS:

SNACKS   FAT   PRTN CARB

                                                     CALS:

NOTES: **TOTALS**
                                                     FAT   PRTN CARB

I DRANK _______________ **WATER**   **GOALS**
MY **PEE** WAS _______________   FAT   PRTN CARB
I HAD _______________ **ENERGY**
MY **MENTAL CLARITY** WAS _______________
I SLEPT _______ HOURS AND FELT _______________
MY **EXERCISE** WAS _______________
AND I DID IT FOR _______ MINUTES AND FELT _______________

CURRENT MOTIVATIONS: _______________

____

____

____

CURRENT SUCCESSES: _______________

____

____

____

LEARNING CURVES: _______________

____

____

____

NEXT WEEK'S PLAN: _______________

____

____

____

DATE   DAY #

BREAKFAST   FAT   PRTN CARB

                                               CALS:

LUNCH   FAT   PRTN CARB

                                               CALS:

DINNER   FAT   PRTN CARB

                                               CALS:

SNACKS   FAT   PRTN CARB

                                               CALS:

NOTES: **TOTALS**
                                               FAT   PRTN CARB

I DRANK _______________ **WATER**   **GOALS**
MY **PEE** WAS _______________   FAT   PRTN CARB
I HAD _______________ **ENERGY**
MY **MENTAL CLARITY** WAS _______________
I **SLEPT** _______ HOURS AND FELT _______
MY **EXERCISE** WAS _______________
AND I DID IT FOR _______ MINUTES AND FELT _______

DATE   DAY #

START WEIGHT: NOW WEIGHT: GOAL WEIGHT:

CURRENT MOTIVATIONS: _______________
____
____
____

CURRENT SUCCESSES: _______________
____
____
____

LEARNING CURVES: _______________
____
____
____

NEXT WEEK'S PLAN: _______________
____
____
____

WEEK 10

WEEK BEGINNING: **CURRENT WEIGHT:**

ARE YOU HAVING FUN?

Lets see where you can go from here!

DATE   **DAY #**

BREAKFAST   FAT   PRTN CARB

                                             CALS:

LUNCH   FAT   PRTN CARB

                                             CALS:

DINNER   FAT   PRTN CARB

                                             CALS:

SNACKS   FAT   PRTN CARB

                                             CALS:

NOTES: **TOTALS**
                                             FAT   PRTN CARB

I DRANK   **WATER**   **GOALS**
MY **PEE** WAS   FAT   PRTN CARB
I HAD   **ENERGY**
MY **MENTAL CLARITY** WAS
I **SLEPT**   HOURS AND FELT
MY **EXERCISE** WAS
AND I DID IT FOR   MINUTES AND FELT

DATE   DAY #

START WEIGHT: NOW WEIGHT: GOAL WEIGHT:

CURRENT MOTIVATIONS: _________________

____

____

____

CURRENT SUCCESSES: _________________

____

____

____

LEARNING CURVES: _________________

____

____

____

NEXT WEEK'S PLAN: _________________

____

____

____

DATE   DAY #

BREAKFAST   FAT   PRTN   CARB

CALS:

LUNCH   FAT   PRTN   CARB

CALS:

DINNER   FAT   PRTN   CARB

CALS:

SNACKS   FAT   PRTN   CARB

CALS:

NOTES: **TOTALS**

                    FAT   PRTN   CARB

I DRANK _______ **WATER**   **GOALS**

MY **PEE** WAS _______   FAT   PRTN   CARB

I HAD _______ **ENERGY**

MY **MENTAL CLARITY** WAS _______

I **SLEPT** _______ HOURS AND FELT _______

MY **EXERCISE** WAS _______

AND I DID IT FOR _______ MINUTES AND FELT _______

DATE   **DAY #**

START WEIGHT: **NOW WEIGHT:**   **GOAL WEIGHT:**

CURRENT MOTIVATIONS: _______________
____
____
____

CURRENT SUCCESSES: _______________
____
____
____

LEARNING CURVES: _______________
____
____
____

NEXT WEEK'S PLAN: _______________
____
____
____

DATE   DAY #

BREAKFAST   FAT   PRTN CARB

                                           CALS:

LUNCH   FAT   PRTN CARB

                                           CALS:

DINNER   FAT   PRTN CARB

                                           CALS:

SNACKS   FAT   PRTN CARB

                                           CALS:

NOTES: **TOTALS**
                                           FAT   PRTN CARB

I DRANK _______________ **WATER**   **GOALS**
MY **PEE** WAS _______________   FAT   PRTN CARB
I HAD _______________ **ENERGY**
MY **MENTAL CLARITY** WAS _______________
I **SLEPT** _______ HOURS AND FELT _______________
MY **EXERCISE** WAS _______________
AND I DID IT FOR _______ MINUTES AND FELT _______________

CURRENT MOTIVATIONS: _____________________

____

____

____

CURRENT SUCCESSES: _____________________

____

____

____

LEARNING CURVES: _____________________

____

____

____

NEXT WEEK'S PLAN: _____________________

____

____

____

DATE   **DAY #**

BREAKFAST   FAT   PRTN   CARB

CALS:

LUNCH   FAT   PRTN   CARB

CALS:

DINNER   FAT   PRTN   CARB

CALS:

SNACKS   FAT   PRTN   CARB

CALS:

NOTES: **TOTALS**
                                                 FAT   PRTN   CARB

I DRANK ________________ **WATER**   **GOALS**
MY **PEE** WAS   FAT   PRTN   CARB
I HAD ________________ **ENERGY**
MY **MENTAL CLARITY** WAS
I **SLEPT** ______ HOURS AND FELT
MY **EXERCISE** WAS
AND I DID IT FOR ______ MINUTES AND FELT

CURRENT MOTIVATIONS: ___________________
____
____
____

CURRENT SUCCESSES: ___________________
____
____
____

LEARNING CURVES: ___________________
____
____
____

NEXT WEEK'S PLAN: ___________________
____
____
____

DATE   **DAY #**

BREAKFAST   FAT   PRTN   CARB

                                                     CALS:

LUNCH   FAT   PRTN   CARB

                                                     CALS:

DINNER   FAT   PRTN   CARB

                                                     CALS:

SNACKS   FAT   PRTN   CARB

                                                     CALS:

NOTES: **TOTALS**
                                                     FAT   PRTN   CARB

I DRANK ________________ **WATER**   **GOALS**
MY **PEE** WAS   FAT   PRTN   CARB
I HAD ________________ **ENERGY**
MY **MENTAL CLARITY** WAS
I SLEPT ______ HOURS AND FELT
MY **EXERCISE** WAS
AND I DID IT FOR ______ MINUTES AND FELT

DATE   DAY #

START WEIGHT: NOW WEIGHT: GOAL WEIGHT:

CURRENT MOTIVATIONS: _______________

____

____

____

CURRENT SUCCESSES: _________________

____

____

____

LEARNING CURVES: ___________________

____

____

____

NEXT WEEK'S PLAN: __________________

____

____

____

DATE   DAY #

BREAKFAST   FAT   PRTN CARB

                                                 CALS:

LUNCH   FAT   PRTN CARB

                                                 CALS:

DINNER   FAT   PRTN CARB

                                                 CALS:

SNACKS   FAT   PRTN CARB

                                                 CALS:

NOTES: **TOTALS**
                                                 FAT   PRTN CARB

I DRANK _______________ **WATER**   **GOALS**
MY **PEE** WAS   FAT   PRTN CARB
I HAD _______________ **ENERGY**
MY **MENTAL CLARITY** WAS
I **SLEPT** _______ HOURS AND FELT
MY **EXERCISE** WAS
AND I DID IT FOR _______ MINUTES AND FELT

CURRENT MOTIVATIONS: _______________
____
____
____

CURRENT SUCCESSES: _______________
____
____
____

LEARNING CURVES: _______________
____
____
____

NEXT WEEK'S PLAN: _______________
____
____
____

DATE   DAY #

BREAKFAST   FAT   PRTN CARB

                                                 CALS:

LUNCH   FAT   PRTN CARB

                                                 CALS:

DINNER   FAT   PRTN CARB

                                                 CALS:

SNACKS   FAT   PRTN CARB

                                                 CALS:

NOTES: **TOTALS**
                                                 FAT   PRTN CARB

I DRANK   **WATER**   **GOALS**
MY **PEE** WAS   FAT   PRTN CARB
I HAD   **ENERGY**
MY **MENTAL CLARITY** WAS
I **SLEPT**   HOURS AND FELT
MY **EXERCISE** WAS
AND I DID IT FOR   MINUTES AND FELT

DATE   DAY #

START WEIGHT: NOW WEIGHT: GOAL WEIGHT:

CURRENT MOTIVATIONS: _______________________

____

____

____

CURRENT SUCCESSES: _________________________

____

____

____

LEARNING CURVES: ___________________________

____

____

____

NEXT WEEK'S PLAN: __________________________

____

____

____

WEEK 11

WEEK BEGINNING: **CURRENT WEIGHT:**

FAVORITE KETO MOMENT?

Butter looks great on you!

DATE   DAY #

BREAKFAST   FAT   PRTN CARB

                                     CALS:

LUNCH   FAT   PRTN CARB

                                     CALS:

DINNER   FAT   PRTN CARB

                                     CALS:

SNACKS   FAT   PRTN CARB

                                     CALS:

NOTES: **TOTALS**
                                     FAT   PRTN CARB

                              GOALS
I DRANK ______________ **WATER**   FAT   PRTN CARB
MY **PEE** WAS
I HAD ______________ **ENERGY**
MY **MENTAL CLARITY** WAS
I **SLEPT** ______ HOURS AND FELT
MY **EXERCISE** WAS
AND I DID IT FOR ______ MINUTES AND FELT

DATE   DAY #

START WEIGHT: NOW WEIGHT: GOAL WEIGHT:

CURRENT MOTIVATIONS: _______________

____

____

____

CURRENT SUCCESSES: _________________

____

____

____

LEARNING CURVES: ___________________

____

____

____

NEXT WEEK'S PLAN: __________________

____

____

____

DATE   **DAY #**

BREAKFAST   FAT PRTN CARB

                                            CALS:

LUNCH   FAT PRTN CARB

                                            CALS:

DINNER   FAT PRTN CARB

                                            CALS:

SNACKS   FAT PRTN CARB

                                            CALS:

NOTES: **TOTALS**
                                            FAT PRTN CARB

I DRANK _______________ **WATER**   **GOALS**
MY **PEE** WAS   FAT PRTN CARB
I HAD _______________ **ENERGY**
MY **MENTAL CLARITY** WAS
I **SLEPT** _______ HOURS AND FELT
MY **EXERCISE** WAS
AND I DID IT FOR _______ MINUTES AND FELT

DATE   DAY #

START WEIGHT: NOW WEIGHT: GOAL WEIGHT:

CURRENT MOTIVATIONS: ___________________
____
____
____

CURRENT SUCCESSES: _____________________
____
____
____

LEARNING CURVES: _______________________
____
____
____

NEXT WEEK'S PLAN: ______________________
____
____
____

DATE   **DAY #**

BREAKFAST   FAT   PRTN CARB

CALS:

LUNCH   FAT   PRTN CARB

CALS:

DINNER   FAT   PRTN CARB

CALS:

SNACKS   FAT   PRTN CARB

CALS:

NOTES:

TOTALS

FAT   PRTN CARB

GOALS

FAT   PRTN CARB

I DRANK ____________ **WATER**

MY **PEE** WAS ____________

I HAD ____________ **ENERGY**

MY **MENTAL CLARITY** WAS ____________

I SLEPT ____ HOURS AND FELT ____________

MY **EXERCISE** WAS ____________

AND I DID IT FOR ____ MINUTES AND FELT ____________

DATE   **DAY #**

BREAKFAST   FAT   PRTN CARB

                                                 CALS:

LUNCH   FAT   PRTN CARB

                                                 CALS:

DINNER   FAT   PRTN CARB

                                                 CALS:

SNACKS   FAT   PRTN CARB

                                                 CALS:

NOTES: **TOTALS**
                                                 FAT   PRTN CARB

I DRANK ________________ **WATER**   **GOALS**
MY **PEE** WAS   FAT   PRTN CARB
I HAD ________________ **ENERGY**
MY **MENTAL CLARITY** WAS
I **SLEPT** ________ HOURS AND FELT
MY **EXERCISE** WAS
AND I DID IT FOR ________ MINUTES AND FELT

DATE ________________________ DAY # ____________

START WEIGHT: __________ NOW WEIGHT: __________ GOAL WEIGHT: __________

CURRENT MOTIVATIONS: _________________

____

____

____

CURRENT SUCCESSES: _________________

____

____

____

LEARNING CURVES: _________________

____

____

____

NEXT WEEK'S PLAN: _________________

____

____

____

DATE   DAY #

BREAKFAST   FAT   PRTN   CARB

CALS:

LUNCH   FAT   PRTN   CARB

CALS:

DINNER   FAT   PRTN   CARB

CALS:

SNACKS   FAT   PRTN   CARB

CALS:

NOTES: **TOTALS**

FAT   PRTN   CARB

I DRANK   **WATER**   **GOALS**

MY **PEE** WAS   FAT   PRTN   CARB

I HAD   **ENERGY**

MY **MENTAL CLARITY** WAS

I **SLEPT**   HOURS AND FELT

MY **EXERCISE** WAS

AND I DID IT FOR   MINUTES AND FELT

DATE   **DAY #**

START WEIGHT: **NOW WEIGHT:**   **GOAL WEIGHT:**

CURRENT MOTIVATIONS: ___________________
____
____
____

CURRENT SUCCESSES: ___________________
____
____
____

LEARNING CURVES: ___________________
____
____
____

NEXT WEEK'S PLAN: ___________________
____
____
____

DATE   **DAY #**

BREAKFAST   FAT PRTN CARB

CALS:

LUNCH   FAT PRTN CARB

CALS:

DINNER   FAT PRTN CARB

CALS:

SNACKS   FAT PRTN CARB

CALS:

NOTES: **TOTALS**

FAT PRTN CARB

GOALS

FAT PRTN CARB

I DRANK __________ **WATER**

MY **PEE** WAS __________

I HAD __________ **ENERGY**

MY **MENTAL CLARITY** WAS __________

I **SLEPT** __________ HOURS AND FELT __________

MY **EXERCISE** WAS __________

AND I DID IT FOR __________ MINUTES AND FELT __________

DATE   **DAY #**

START WEIGHT: **NOW WEIGHT:**   **GOAL WEIGHT:**

CURRENT MOTIVATIONS: _______________
____
____
____

CURRENT SUCCESSES: _______________
____
____
____

LEARNING CURVES: _______________
____
____
____

NEXT WEEK'S PLAN: _______________
____
____
____

DATE   DAY #

BREAKFAST   FAT   PRTN CARB

CALS:

LUNCH   FAT   PRTN CARB

CALS:

DINNER   FAT   PRTN CARB

CALS:

SNACKS   FAT   PRTN CARB

CALS:

NOTES: **TOTALS**
                                FAT   PRTN CARB

I DRANK ________________ **WATER**   **GOALS**
MY **PEE** WAS   FAT   PRTN CARB
I HAD ________________ **ENERGY**
MY **MENTAL CLARITY** WAS
I **SLEPT** ______ HOURS AND FELT
MY **EXERCISE** WAS
AND I DID IT FOR ______ MINUTES AND FELT

DATE   **DAY #**

START WEIGHT: **NOW WEIGHT:**   **GOAL WEIGHT:**

CURRENT MOTIVATIONS: _________________________

____

____

____

CURRENT SUCCESSES: _________________________

____

____

____

LEARNING CURVES: _________________________

____

____

____

NEXT WEEK'S PLAN: _________________________

____

____

____

WEEK 12

WEEK BEGINNING: **CURRENT WEIGHT:**

READY FOR WHAT'S NEXT?

Congrats, you're fat adapted!

DATE   **DAY #**

BREAKFAST   FAT   PRTN CARB

                                                       CALS:

LUNCH   FAT   PRTN CARB

                                                       CALS:

DINNER   FAT   PRTN CARB

                                                       CALS:

SNACKS   FAT   PRTN CARB

                                                       CALS:

NOTES: **TOTALS**
                                                       FAT   PRTN CARB

I DRANK ________________ **WATER**   **GOALS**
MY **PEE** WAS ________________   FAT   PRTN CARB
I HAD ________________ **ENERGY**
MY **MENTAL CLARITY** WAS ________________
I SLEPT ________ HOURS AND FELT ________________
MY **EXERCISE** WAS ________________
AND I DID IT FOR ________ MINUTES AND FELT ________________

DATE   **DAY #**

START WEIGHT: **NOW WEIGHT:**   **GOAL WEIGHT:**

CURRENT MOTIVATIONS: _______________________
____
____
____

CURRENT SUCCESSES: _______________________
____
____
____

LEARNING CURVES: _______________________
____
____
____

NEXT WEEK'S PLAN: _______________________
____
____

DATE   **DAY #**

BREAKFAST   FAT   PRTN CARB

CALS:

LUNCH   FAT   PRTN CARB

CALS:

DINNER   FAT   PRTN CARB

CALS:

SNACKS   FAT   PRTN CARB

CALS:

NOTES:

TOTALS		
FAT	PRTN	CARB

I DRANK ____________________ **WATER**

MY **PEE** WAS

GOALS		
FAT	PRTN	CARB

I HAD ________________ **ENERGY**

MY **MENTAL CLARITY** WAS

I SLEPT ______ HOURS AND FELT

MY **EXERCISE** WAS

AND I DID IT FOR ______ MINUTES AND FELT

DATE   **DAY #**

START WEIGHT: **NOW WEIGHT:**   **GOAL WEIGHT:**

CURRENT MOTIVATIONS: _______________________

____

____

____

CURRENT SUCCESSES: _______________________

____

____

____

LEARNING CURVES: _______________________

____

____

____

NEXT WEEK'S PLAN: _______________________

____

____

____

DATE   DAY #

BREAKFAST   FAT   PRTN CARB

                                  CALS:

LUNCH   FAT   PRTN CARB

                                  CALS:

DINNER   FAT   PRTN CARB

                                  CALS:

SNACKS   FAT   PRTN CARB

                                  CALS:

NOTES: **TOTALS**
                                  FAT   PRTN CARB

I DRANK   **WATER**   **GOALS**
MY **PEE** WAS   FAT   PRTN CARB
I HAD   **ENERGY**
MY **MENTAL CLARITY** WAS
I **SLEPT**   HOURS AND FELT
MY **EXERCISE** WAS
AND I DID IT FOR   MINUTES AND FELT

DATE   DAY #

START WEIGHT: NOW WEIGHT: GOAL WEIGHT:

CURRENT MOTIVATIONS: ______________________

____

____

____

CURRENT SUCCESSES: ______________________

____

____

____

LEARNING CURVES: ______________________

____

____

____

NEXT WEEK'S PLAN: ______________________

____

____

____

DATE   DAY #

BREAKFAST   FAT   PRTN CARB

                                             CALS:

LUNCH   FAT   PRTN CARB

                                             CALS:

DINNER   FAT   PRTN CARB

                                             CALS:

SNACKS   FAT   PRTN CARB

                                             CALS:

NOTES: **TOTALS**
                                             FAT   PRTN CARB

I DRANK _______________ **WATER**   **GOALS**
MY **PEE** WAS   FAT   PRTN CARB
I HAD _______________ **ENERGY**
MY **MENTAL CLARITY** WAS
I **SLEPT** _______ HOURS AND FELT
MY **EXERCISE** WAS
AND I DID IT FOR _______ MINUTES AND FELT

DATE   DAY #

START WEIGHT: NOW WEIGHT: GOAL WEIGHT:

CURRENT MOTIVATIONS: _________________
____
____
____

CURRENT SUCCESSES: _________________
____
____
____

LEARNING CURVES: _________________
____
____
____

NEXT WEEK'S PLAN: _________________
____
____
____

DATE   **DAY #**

BREAKFAST   FAT   PRTN CARB

                                                 CALS:

LUNCH   FAT   PRTN CARB

                                                 CALS:

DINNER   FAT   PRTN CARB

                                                 CALS:

SNACKS   FAT   PRTN CARB

                                                 CALS:

NOTES: **TOTALS**
                                                 FAT   PRTN CARB

I DRANK   **WATER**   **GOALS**
MY **PEE** WAS   FAT   PRTN CARB
I HAD   **ENERGY**
MY **MENTAL CLARITY** WAS
I **SLEPT**   HOURS AND FELT
MY **EXERCISE** WAS
AND I DID IT FOR   MINUTES AND FELT

DATE   **DAY #**

START WEIGHT: **NOW WEIGHT:**   **GOAL WEIGHT:**

CURRENT MOTIVATIONS: ___________________
____
____
____

CURRENT SUCCESSES: ___________________
____
____
____

LEARNING CURVES: ___________________
____
____
____

NEXT WEEK'S PLAN: ___________________
____
____
____

DATE   **DAY #**

BREAKFAST   FAT   PRTN CARB

                                           CALS:

LUNCH   FAT   PRTN CARB

                                           CALS:

DINNER   FAT   PRTN CARB

                                           CALS:

SNACKS   FAT   PRTN CARB

                                           CALS:

NOTES: **TOTALS**
                                           FAT   PRTN CARB

I DRANK   **WATER**   **GOALS**
MY **PEE** WAS   FAT   PRTN CARB
I HAD   **ENERGY**

MY **MENTAL CLARITY** WAS

I **SLEPT**   HOURS AND FELT

MY **EXERCISE** WAS

AND I DID IT FOR   MINUTES AND FELT

DATE   DAY #

START WEIGHT: NOW WEIGHT: GOAL WEIGHT:

CURRENT MOTIVATIONS: ______________________
____
____
____

CURRENT SUCCESSES: ______________________
____
____
____

LEARNING CURVES: ______________________
____
____
____

NEXT WEEK'S PLAN: ______________________
____
____
____

DATE   DAY #

BREAKFAST   FAT   PRTN CARB

                                        CALS:

LUNCH   FAT   PRTN CARB

                                        CALS:

DINNER   FAT   PRTN CARB

                                        CALS:

SNACKS   FAT   PRTN CARB

                                        CALS:

NOTES: **TOTALS**
                                        FAT   PRTN CARB

I DRANK ________________ **WATER**   **GOALS**
MY **PEE** WAS ________________   FAT   PRTN CARB
I HAD ________________ **ENERGY**
MY **MENTAL CLARITY** WAS ________________
I **SLEPT** ______ HOURS AND FELT ________________
MY **EXERCISE** WAS ________________
AND I DID IT FOR ______ MINUTES AND FELT ________________

DATE   DAY #

START WEIGHT: NOW WEIGHT: GOAL WEIGHT:

CURRENT MOTIVATIONS: __________________

____

____

____

CURRENT SUCCESSES: __________________

____

____

____

LEARNING CURVES: __________________

____

____

____

NEXT WEEK'S PLAN: __________________

____

____

____

9 781730 895555